ABOUT GINSENG

How ginseng has been used as a panacea for thousands of years in the East; its natural habitat, and cultivation of the root throughout the world; some scientific evidence of its properties; its effect on the ageing process; the different forms available, where to buy it, and dosage; its future in the field of medicine.

108/110 Charing Cross Road,

London WC2

Tel: 01-240 0636/7.

Telex: 299340

KOREAN GINSENG CENTRE

LOTTE TRADING (UK) CO. LTD.

ABOUT GINSENG
The Magical Herb of the East

by

STEPHEN FULDER, M.A., Ph.D

THORSONS PUBLISHERS LIMITED
Wellingborough, Northamptonshire

First published January 1976
Second Impression July 1976
Third Impression March 1977
Fourth Impression June 1977
Fifth Impression March 1978

ISBN 0 7225 0327 X

Printed and bound in Great Britain
by Richard Clay (The Chaucer Press), Ltd
Bungay, Suffolk

CONTENTS

Page

Chapter

1. Brother of Soma — 7
2. Ginseng and Herbal Medicine
      in China — 13
3. The Root that Hides from Man — 22
4. Some Scientific Evidence — 29
5. The Elixir? — 42
6. How to Take Ginseng — 50
7. Ginseng and Traditional
      Medicine Today — 58

DEDICATION

To Dorothy Herschfeld

ACKNOWLEDGEMENTS

I would like to acknowledge Pharmaton S.A. for helping me to obtain scientific papers and Joseph Needham for the use of his library on China. I thank Helen Varley for comments on the manuscript. Of course I would also like to acknowledge the help of ginseng, without which this book would have taken much longer.

CHAPTER ONE
BROTHER OF SOMA

Of all the multitude of plant medicines known, ginseng seems to be one of the most interesting. It is the only plant which, for thousands of years, has been consistently claimed to be a panacea – a universal remedy. Its full name, *Panax ginseng*, illustrates this, for Panax, like panacea, comes from the Greek work for 'all-healing'. No other plant is used so widely in the Orient for so many diseases and ailments. The Chinese, whose traditional medicine is without doubt one of the most sophisticated medical systems known to man, rely heavily on ginseng both as an essential tonic and restorative and as a regular part of the complex battery of plants compounded for the treatment of serious diseases.

Ginseng is unique because it is the plant used most widely in combating some of the degenerative conditions and loss of vitality that accompanies ageing, and, not surprisingly, a special reverence for it has developed over the ages. It is embodied in many stories and legends; in fact, it could be said that no other plant has such an extensive mythology.

There are other unique features of ginseng which are important for our point of view: it seems to be the only plant which can so clearly demonstrate the philosophy behind traditional healing, and certainly no other has been the subject of such extensive scientific research yielding such puzzling and paradoxical conclusions. Finally, it is strikingly obvious that there is no other medicinal plant which is used so extensively in one half of the world, and ignored so completely in the other half.

Panax ginseng is the botanical name of a shrub of the family *Araliaceae*. It grows deep inside forest areas, preferring a moist shaded environment. It has an array of leaves, usually five, at the end of a long stalk which may be a metre high. Small lilac flowers appear in the early summer, and red and black berries in autumn. The medicinal part is the root which is white, branched and fleshy, and covered in tendrils. There are various species and varieties of the plant. *Panax ginseng* grows in China, Korea and Eastern U.S.S.R., and *Panax japonicus* in Japan. *Panax pseudoginseng* and related varieties can be found in the Himalayas of India and Nepal, and *Panax quinquefolium* grows in America. The root of ginseng is often likened to a man in shape. This has generated its Chinese name 'ginseng', meaning 'man-like', and also the Iroquois Indian name for it, 'garentoquen', meaning the shape of a man's thighs. The mandrake root is also man-shaped, and because of certain similar legends, such as that the plant cries when drawn from the soil, the two plants are sometimes confused. They are in fact completely unrelated.

Ginseng as Legend

A medicinal plant as important as ginseng is more than just a medicine to the people who use it. It is a veritable gift from the benign divine powers.

Extensive ritual surrounds the gathering, planting, storing, preparing and consuming of the root. The many legends have given rise to many names. One story describes how the village Shantan, in Shensi province, was troubled for many nights by a groaning and wailing somewhere behind the village. Although much afraid of this strange occurrence, the villagers organized an expedition one night to discover the source of the unearthly cries. They took torches and staves and eventually localized the sound to a large bush about a mile away. They dug up the bush and found underneath a huge root, of the shape and size of a man. The crying stopped. From this the root became known as 'spirit of the earth' (*ti ching*).

Ginseng is derived from the words *jen sheng*, which, in addition to 'man-like', mean 'like-the-constellation-of-Orion'. Orion is traditionally shaped like a man, and is also the constellation which has astrological influence over ginseng. Other names of ginseng are: blood-like (*hsueh shen*), human bridle (*jen hsien*), devil cover (*kuei kai*), magical herb (*shen tshao*), and the more down-to-earth name, the-regenerating-elixir-that-banishes-wrinkles-from-the-face (*tson mien huntan*). The Koreans call the herb Korean phoenix (*Poughwang*).

The Man-like Root

The Chinese undoubtedly revered ginseng above any other plant. This is reflected in the fabulous prices that were paid for it during the imperial times. An old root, cured properly and of the best quality would fetch much more than its weight in gold. The most cherished roots were those with a man-like shape. The equivalent of hundreds of dollars would be paid for such a root, giving rise to the sarcastic epithet in Manchuria: 'Eat ginseng and ruin yourself.' It was believed that the power of a plant to cure a certain part of the body was reflected in some way in its form. Thus a ginseng root that was shaped like a man was believed to have greater curative powers for the whole body, and particularly for the restoration of male potency.

Manchuria is the traditional home of the most famous wild ginseng. The Manchurians boast that 'the weeds of their country are the choice drugs of the Chinese'. It is often mentioned that one Chinese Emperor set out to war in order to capture ginseng-growing land, and it is certainly true that in 1709 the Emperor sent 10,000 Tartars to search for ginseng, ordering that each soldier should give him two catties of the best and sell the rest for its weight in silver. The Chinese sometimes used to keep the ginseng in lead-lined boxes, carefully wrapped in silk and tissue paper, for they believed that it had certain 'life-giving radiations' which might be lost in an ordinary container. Such radiations are in fact most unlikely, but it illustrates the reverential and almost sacramental treatment given to the herb.

In China the general opinion was that ginseng was the prince of plants. The most famous Chinese herbalist, and one of the founders of Chinese traditional medicine, the Emperor Shen Nung, put forward a classification of herbs which is recorded in the Shen Nung Pen Tshao Ching, the *Pharmacopoeia of the Heavenly Husbandman*, printed in the second century B.C. Several hundred herbs were listed and classified under three groups according to toxicity, or the power of the drug compared with its safety. Ginseng is at the top of the list of those agents which are beneficial, yet harmless.

Ginseng in India and Korea

China is not the only place where ginseng has been used since ancient times. The Vedas are ancient Indian scriptures which reflect an oral teaching which may be 5000 years old. The Atherva Veda has many hymns describing ways to attain health and fulfilment. One hymn descibes ginseng as, 'the root which is dug from the earth and which strengthens the nerves'. It continues: 'the strength of the horse, the mule, the goat, the ram, moreover the strength of the bull it bestows on him. This herb will make thee so full of lusty strength that thou shalt, when excited, exhale heat as a thing on fire.'

The hymn then describes the herb as 'brother of Soma'. Soma is the legendary life-giving plant of India, an elixir which was worshipped and offered in sacrifices. If ginseng is the brother of Soma, it must also have appeared to have unearthly power. On the other hand, ginseng is not a feature of the Ayurvedic medical system which developed out of the Vedas. This may be because the plant later became unavailable in India.

A Story from Korea

Ginseng is mentioned in Ezekiel (27:17) as one of the exotic herbs brought from the East. Wherever it grows it has given rise to its own myths. In

Korea it is related how a son and grandson, both very poor, were devotedly looking after an ailing grandfather. One night the grandson couldn't sleep. The candle kept on blowing out. He was suddenly aware that there was no wind to blow out the candle and that there must be a spirit presence in the room. The boy took a needle and thread, and the next time he felt the presence of the spirit he plunged the needle in that direction. The needle disappeared and the boy followed it by means of the unravelling thread. Eventually he found the needle. It was stuck in the ground at the base of a wild ginseng plant. The boy took the plant and brewed a decoction for his grandfather, who recovered. Thus the spirit of the ginseng plant had rewarded the boy for his selfless devotion.

There are many more myths and rituals, some of which will be related when discussing the way ginseng is collected and cultivated, cured and consumed. The essence of the legends is that ginseng has an almost supernatural power for the good of man. We can understand this a little better if we consider the Chinese philosophy of the Tao. The Tao literally means 'the way'. It is the incomprehensible flow of energy of the cosmos which finds its temporary expression in the materials of Nature. Man is one of the materials; he is not at the head of Nature but in unity with Nature, neither more nor less important than any other part. He is also subject to the balanced forces of good and bad. These forces are to be reverently respected. Ginseng represents a beneficial aspect of Nature and is therefore to be treated like a great gift.

CHAPTER TWO

GINSENG AND HERBAL MEDICINE IN CHINA

You exist on plants. Virtually all the food that you eat is either from the plant kingdom, or from animals who eat from the plant kingdom. Moreover, the cigarette you may be smoking, the perfume you may be smelling, the clothes you may be wearing, the chair you may be sitting on, and the very pages of the book you are now reading are derived from one or other plant species. The number of different types of plants in use as medicines is certainly greater than all the plants in use for any other purpose. The Indian system of traditional medicine, the Ayurvedic system, said to date from 3000 B.C., holds that not a single plant in the plant kingdom is useless. Plants are blessed for the help they give. As it says in the Vedas:

> All the many herbs in which the human physicians
>   find a remedy,
> Like mothers assembled let them yield milk
> Unto man, for freedom from harm.

Compare this with the naïve view of herbal remedies held by some practitioners of conventional medicine. Dr Williams, working in China at the turn of the century, writes cynically about Chinese traditional medicine: 'Anything indeed that is thoroughly disgusting in the three kingdoms of Nature is considered good enough for medicinal use.' Dr Williams also appears to have come to the conclusion that almost every plant is useful in medicine, although he refuses to see it as a blessing!

Many plants, such as digitalis, raowolfia, datura and ephedra, are used exclusively for medicines; others – for example, those commonly known as garlic, mint, coffee, banana, caraway and liquorice – are both food and medicine. The variety of plants which act on the human body is so great that it takes a man many years to learn of the medicinal wealth around him, whether he lives in China or Canada.

A Kingly Herb

Chinese traditional medicine is probably the most complicated and esoteric medical system known, and little of it is properly understood in the West. We can return to the *Pharmacopoeia of the Heavenly Husbandman* to find an interesting clue to the way herbs were used in China. Those which are mild in effect and not harmful even in large doses are the 'kingly' herbs. The second group, more powerful herbs which are rather more toxic, are called 'ministerial'. The lowest group, called merely 'adjutant', are the highly powerful herbs which are at the same time dangerous.

The essential point is that the mildest herbs are the most important and of the first rank, while the really powerful herbs are last-resort drugs to be used only when the others fail. This is of course the opposite position to that of Western (allopathic) medicine, which regards the powerful drugs as the mainstay of medicine, and the mild drugs as accessories of little significance.

The basic principle of Chinese traditional

medicine is to attempt to maintain the body in peak health. If the body is healthy it will automatically be more resistant to disease, just as a car which is tuned and serviced will be much less likely to undergo a serious breakdown. Therefore the primary task of the traditional practitioners is to ensure the continuing health of the people they look after, and secondarily to treat diseases. A Chinese doctor used to be paid by his patients only when they were in good health. When they became ill the doctor was not paid, because he had failed to keep his patient healthy. It is fair to say that while the focus of traditional medicine is on health, the focus of allopathic medicine is on sickness. We can now see why the mild herbs are the most important, the 'kingly' ones. They are the first and primary weapon of the practitioners in health maintenance, and ginseng is chief of all the kingly herbs.

Superimposed on this fundamental concept are complex instructions which relate different herbs to different ailments affecting parts of the body. One further aspect of Chinese philosophy is that Nature is composed of balanced forces of positive and negative, male and female, active and passive. The former is termed 'yang', the latter 'yin'. A basic source of ill health is an imbalance of the two forces within the body. Herbs can be taken to correct the imbalance before it leads to disease. Ginseng is notable as the most 'yang' of all the known herbs.

Ginseng is present as a constituent of nearly every tonic and restorative used by the traditional doctors. A common general tonic, for example, is made up as:

Ginseng extract	2 parts
Root of *Atractylis lancea*	2 parts
'Fou ling' (*Pachyma cocos*)	2 parts
Liquorice root (*Glycyrrhiza glabra*)	1 part

Moreover, ginseng is a component of nearly every preparation for more serious diseases — for example, smallpox, fevers, circulatory and nervous diseases. Here we find elaborate mixtures of plants and substances, both mild and powerful, medicinal and more or less magical. For example, the 'Seven Precious' powder for wound healing contains:

> Dragon's bone and blood
> Elephant skin
> Ginseng root
> *Gimura pinnatifidia*
> Frankincense (Boswellia)
> Myrrh (*Commiphoa myrrha*)
> Laka wood.

Chieh-pin Chang (A.D. 960) listed some 500 medicinal formulae containing ginseng, prescribed for nearly every type of disease, with few exceptions.

Chinese Medicine Today

Traditional medicine in China is not an archaic code of instructions present only in old books. It is a living system which is used today in combination with allopathic medicine in a unique synthesis. For example, in the teaching hospitals of Peking, surgery will be carried out in the Western manner with highly advanced equipment, but the anaesthetist may use acupuncture instead of pentothal, and herbal preparations will be used for pre- and post-operative treatment. Ginseng is nearly always present in these preparations to increase the resistance of the patient, protect his system against shock during the operation, and increase his vitality during post-operative recovery.

The impetus for this novel approach seems to have come from Chairman Mao himself ('the past must serve the present') and the cultural revolution. A rural health system has been instituted in China in which doctors, trained in the major teaching hospitals, then spread out to the rural areas and in turn train health workers at the village level. These famous 'barefoot doctors' teach disease prevention, sanitation and first aid. Deadly diseases such as cholera and smallpox have been completely eliminated in China in a remarkably short time by this system.

At the same time knowledge of traditional medicine has spread in the opposite direction — from the villages to the cities where it is now studied at research institutes. Here it is investigated in an open-minded way, with full awareness of ancient medical principles. The result has been most successful, for in that way the Chinese can call upon the experience of 4000 years of experiment and knowledge of herbs. Acupuncture, the ancient technique of anaesthesia and healing, is similarly encouraged. The important point is that it works, whether or not it conforms to the current scientific theories. If Chinese herbal medicine is judged with a 'proof of the pudding' attitude, one cannot fail to be impressed. As an eminent specialist remarked on a visit to China: 'We may look forward to a whole range of new drugs of enormous potential for medicine in general.' Ginseng is the first of these.

The Uses of Ginseng

The *Pharmacopoeia of the Heavenly Husbandman* states that ginseng is a 'tonic to the five viscera, quieting the animal spirits, strengthening the soul, allaying fear, expelling evil effluvia, brightening the eyes, opening the heart, benefiting the understanding, and if taken for some time, it will invigorate the body and prolong life.'

More modern pharmacopoeias (manuals of medicines) echo this earliest record. They state that ginseng prevents tiredness, headaches, exhaustion, amnesia, and the debilitating effects of old age, and confirm that it is a useful adjunct in the treatment of tuberculosis, diabetes, diseases of the heart, kidneys, nervous and circulatory systems; moreover, it is said to prevent declining potency in older men. In a word, it is a powerful restorative and curative agent. We will examine the effects of ginseng in detail in subsequent chapters, but it is clear that if even part of these attributes can be proved, it will have earned its reputation as a panacea.

A Stimulant

It is traditionally held in all the countries which use ginseng that it is a stimulant and can increase the resistance of the body. The sick take it to restore strength. Chinese soldiers carry it on to the battlefield to prevent the effects of stress and shock if they are wounded and to sustain them until they can be brought to the field hospital. Soldiers also use it as a stimulant for sentry duty, and it is recorded that the North Vietnamese used it extensively in the recent war. Ginseng was taken by Russian astronauts to help them resist infections and disease in their space capsule. This protective use of the plant is precisely within the spirit of traditional medicine.

The stimulant action of ginseng is graphically described by Father Jartoux, the French priest who brought it to the notice of the Royal Society of London, by means of a letter published in 1714. He was riding with the emperor until he was so exhausted that he could hardly keep himself from falling off his horse. The Emperor gave him half a root of ginseng. He chewed it, whereupon he forgot all about his tiredness and carried on full of energy.

The plant can save the lives of seriously ill patients by giving them the energy, vitality and stamina to fight the disease. The Chinese have described many cases in which the sick have been practically *in articulo mortis* when, upon administration of good quality ginseng root, they have been sufficiently revived to carry on items of business. It is a common practice in China to give ginseng to someone on his deathbed in order to give him the power to receive his family and arrange his affairs before departing this world. As Dr Porter Smith noticed: 'Several cases in which life would seem to have been at least prolonged by taking doses of the drug so as to allow intelligent disposal of property, indicate that some positive efficacy of a sustaining character does really exist in this species.'

Ginseng has also earned itself a reputation as an aphrodisiac (a drug which stimulates sexual desire). In fact, *Encyclopaedia Britannica* uses ginseng as an example of a 'genuine' aphrodisiac. The quotation from the Atherva Veda: 'The strength of the horse, the mule, the goat . . .' is so explicit concerning the aphrodisiac effects of ginseng that in the classic translation it is modestly put into Latin rather than English like the rest of the hymns. In actual fact, the extent of its use as an aphrodisiac is uncertain. While the Emperors are known to have consumed much ginseng at court, it cannot be established whether they took it as an aphrodisiac or as a general stimulant. It may be that its reputation as an aphrodisiac owes much to the fancy of European observers at the Imperial court rather than to fact.

On the other hand, ginseng is without doubt used very widely to combat impotence, especially the decline in virility which occurs with age. So much so, that Dr Jeffreys, in his *Diseases of China*, observes that ginseng is used 'chiefly in cases of matrimonial unproductivity'. He seems to have been struck by the popular use of ginseng for that purpose, rather than by any of its other multitudinous uses. Travellers in China, from Marco Polo onwards, have also been impressed by the virility of the Chinese people of advanced years, and the Chinese themselves readily admit that it is partly the use of ginseng which is responsible.

Long-term Benefits

The herbal tradition of ginseng states explicitly that the more ginseng is taken, the more long-term benefits can be obtained from it. It is recommended that everyone who can afford it should take a course of ginseng every year. The effect is cumulative. The regular use of ginseng, it is stated, will not only increase health and vitality but will also prolong life. Old people are advised to take some every single day to extend their lifespan and to encourage protection from the diseases of old age. If it can be authenticated that it is really a 'regenerative elixir that banishes wrinkles from the face', it will be the first known medicine or drug which would be specifically useful for the aged. We devote a subsequent chapter to this intriguing possibility.

Other Oriental countries which use ginseng as part of their traditional medical system ascribe properties to it which are almost identical. The Materia Indica of 1826, for example, states that ginseng 'nourishes and strengthens the body, stops vomiting, clears the judgement, removes hypochondrias and all nervous affectations, and in a word, gives a vigorous tone to the body even in old age.'

CHAPTER THREE

THE ROOT THAT HIDES FROM MAN

Yet another of the names given to ginseng is 'The Root that Hides from Man'. This is meant literally, for the root prefers a habitat deep within thick forest, in moist, rich and undisturbed soil. It sometimes favours specific trees as neighbours, as this Korean song shows:

> The branches which grow from my stalks are three in number, and the leaves are five by five,
> The back part of the leaves is turned to the sky, and the upper side downward,
> Whoever would find me must look for the Kia tree.

Finding wild ginseng was so difficult that searchers could do little else but pray to the spirits which guard it to favour their quest. In Korea, wild-ginseng gatherers would keep chaste and pure for a week before the expedition, praying continuously to their guardian deity. The team was always a group of ten senior villagers led by 'The Man'. They used a secret sign language during their quest, and would refrain from talking, for they were fearful of incurring the displeasure of the Nature spirits guarding ginseng.

In China it is related that searchers were assisted because the leaves of the ginseng plant would sometimes glow at night. The glow would go out if anyone approached, so the searcher would shoot an arrow at it and come back in daylight to look for the arrow and pull the plant. The glow has led to some extravagant theories concerning supposed radiations from ginseng. Yet it may be unnecessary to look further than those fascinating insects, glow-worms, for an explanation. Glow-worms extinguish their lights when approached, and they may collect on ginseng leaves.

Most of the gathering of wild ginseng in Manchuria used to be done on behalf of the Emperor. The common people had to try poaching, or make do with inferior cultivated or imported roots. It still grows wild in Manchuria, the Ussuri region of the U.S.S.R. and in Korea, but extensive picking and the felling of forests have more or less dried up the supplies of wild ginseng all over the world.

Ginseng Cultivation

The earliest plantations of ginseng were in south-east Manchuria, and in North Korea, and cultivation is still carried out in those places, though the product is entirely for home consumption. Major cultivation areas have developed in Russia and South Korea since World War II. There are United States consular reports which describe how the Russians started their ginseng plantations in South Siberia with young plants worth 120 million dollars which were taken home from North Korea in the aftermath of the war.

Cultivation in South Korea is big business. It is one of that country's major exports and under government monopoly. Yet it is still carried out with ceremony and elaborate preparation. Prayers are said before sowing. The seeds are put into specially prepared germination beds after pre-sowing treatment. After a year or more the seeds germinate and are transplanted into drained loam, well spaced, in beds that have lain fallow for many years, and are at the right inclination to the sun. Straw shades are put over the growing plants to mimic the forest conditions as closely as possible.

The plant grows for five years before it is usable. It is slow growing, and can reach an astonishing age. There is a Russian report of a huge wild root which appears, from the rings around the root top, to be 400 years old. However, experts at the Royal Botanical Gardens in Kew are sceptical about this.

Ginseng in America

Both wild and cultivated ginseng are available in the United States, but the plant is a different species from the Asiatic ginseng and does not have the same medicinal properties. If we turn to the traditional medicine in America, namely that of the American Indians, we find that ginseng is used especially by tribes such as the Menomini, Cherokees and the Creeks, who lived in the mountainous areas of mid-America where the plant grows wild. Although the medicine men used it with perhaps even more ritual, sorcery and spirit guidance than the Taoist healers of China, the medicinal uses were severely limited. The only consistent claims made for it are that it is useful in stomach upsets, digestive failure, ear-ache and sometimes wound healing.

Naturally, ginseng was wildly advertised by the notorious quack doctors of the early white settlers in America, but so was everything else. The official United States Pharmacopoeia during the last century does list ginseng, but only as a stomachic and stimulant, and subsequently it was dropped altogether. The very modest claims made reflect the fact that the American species, like the Himalayan one, does not have anything like the same medicinal value as the real Asiatic *Panax ginseng*.

The ginseng grown in America provides an extraordinary story from an economic and social point of view. It is not commonly known that ginseng digging provided the main source of support for some of the early settlers in America. The enterprise began in Canada where a Jesuit missionary, Father Lafiteau, discovered in 1716 a plant similar to the one described by Father Jartoux in China. Avid collection soon began for despatch to China, which was an unlimited market for ginseng, and boatloads were exported to Canton at a profit so huge that ginseng became second only to the fur trade in profitability.

End of the Canadian Trade
Indiscriminate picking and inadequate preparation of the roots dried up the Canadian trade by 1760. The United States took over, and trade expanded. In 1862, a good year for the trade, 622,761 pounds of dried roots were shipped to Canton and Hong Kong. Fur trappers used to return from the mountains with fur and ginseng, and in fact ginseng trade in America today is still carried out by the fur companies. Entire villages in Kentucky and Wisconsin used to go out into the forest and, with 'mattock and sack', dig for 'seng', as it was known. They sometimes managed to collect bushels of roots in a day. The price rose

and rose. It is recorded in a book on Daniel Boone that he personally collected large amounts of ginseng and purchased more from the white settlers. In the winter of 1787-8 he started up the Ohio in a boat containing nearly *fifteen tons* of ginseng. The boat overturned and he lost it all. Undismayed, he had collected fifteen 'caggs' again by the following autumn.

When wild ginseng became scarce at the end of the nineteenth century, some enterprising farmers attempted cultivation, and a few made a great success of it. However, ginseng is liked by other species besides humans and glow-worms – namely, all kinds of insects, fungi, pests and worms. Virtually the entire American crop was wiped out by 1910, and the Depression finished off many farms. Despite this, some export of ginseng to China continues up to the present day, and ginseng was one of the only exports from America to China during the 1950 to 1960 period.

Has ginseng been grown in Europe? Father Lafiteau sent fresh samples from Canada to France, where they were transplanted without success. The Royal Botanical Gardens in Kew have not attempted to grow it. There is no reason why it should not be grown in Europe and other places, yet there is no report of anyone having done so. Here is a golden opportunity for someone with green fingers!

Ginseng in the Market

The root which is available in shops is never fresh. It has undergone an elaborate process of curing and drying which preserves the essential medicinal components and allows the root to be kept for years without decay or decline in potency. The dried root is hard and brittle and has a strong aromatic bitter-sweet taste, not unlike liquorice.

After carefully digging the root from the earth, the fine outer tendrils are removed and it is washed. Some of the roots are steam cured by a secret process which turns them a deep red colour and gives them a remarkable translucent appearance. Others which are not steamed are yellow and opaque. Slow drying in a sequence of warm rooms at different temperatures for a period of months finally preserves and hardens the root and it is ready for consumption.

The quality of the root varies considerably and this is reflected in the price. First quality is the wild Manchurian 'Imperial' white roots which are hugely expensive and virtually never seen outside China. Second quality are the Chinese and Korean red and white roots, which are now always cultivated. The red roots fetch slightly higher prices. Third quality are the Japanese cultivated roots, which were originally started from Korean imports. Fourth quality, according to the Chinese Materia Medica, are the American white roots of *Panax quinquefolium*.

The high cost has always encouraged fraudulent substitutions of other roots for ginseng; for example, *Campanunoea pilosule*, also called 'Bastard Ginseng' (*tang shen*) in China, and *Adenophora verticillata* (*shashen*) both resemble it. The Chinese relate a traditional method of telling the real from the fake. Two persons are chosen and made to walk four Li (a Li is the Chinese mile). One has a piece of the supposed ginseng in his mouth. If at the end of the walk the person without the root is somewhat out of breath, while the man with the root does not feel in the least bit tired, then the drug is true.

There is another plant which has come into the limelight indirectly as a result of ginseng. The Institute of Biologically Active Substances in Vladivostok, U.S.S.R., attempting to find substitutes for ginseng because of its rarity and its reluctance to take to cultivation, searched through the *Arialaceae* family and discovered that a common thorny shrub called *Eleutherococcus senticosus*, which grows in Siberia, China and Korea, had similarities. Tests showed that the roots as well as the leaves possessed wide-ranging and powerful medicinal properties. Strangely, the plant is not used in traditional medicine and not listed in the ancient herbals. It seems that this plant, sometimes confusingly called 'Siberian ginseng', is a rare example of a case where modern scientific research has added to the traditional storehouse of medicinal herbs.

CHAPTER FOUR

SOME SCIENTIFIC EVIDENCE

Ginseng as a Stimulant

The Chinese herbals and the Chinese medical tradition give only a brief mention to the fact that ginseng is a stimulant and will overcome exhaustion. They concentrate rather on the long-term usage in the restoration of health and vitality. Yet scientific research has shown ginseng to be a powerful short-term stimulant, and this is of great potential interest to Westerners, who are badly in need of a stimulant which does no harm. Ginseng, on the contrary, may be a stimulant which actually is good for you.

Subtle long-term effects on health are difficult to measure with the techniques of modern science, so that research has concentrated more on detecting short-term actions. This has emphasized the stimulant effect of ginseng in the eyes of Westerners, but it must be remembered that the emphasis in traditional and herbal medicine is just the reverse.

Some of the earliest experiments on this stimulant action were carried out on mice by Professor Brekhman, head of the Institute of Biologically Active Substances in Vladivostok. He devised a swimming test to see if ginseng could increase stamina. Mice are put into water, where they swim until they are exhausted. They are allowed to rest, and then made to swim a second time. Professor Brekhman showed that mice given ginseng were able to swim nearly twice as long before they were exhausted.

The same experiment has been repeated in many parts of the world, with the same result. A European laboratory has recently demonstrated that even if the mice are given doses of ginseng similar to the normal human doses, their increase in stamina is still quite noticeable. The ginseng effect is cumulative. If mice are given ginseng continuously for a month they can then regularly swim for twice as long as those mice not given ginseng.

Russian scientists have examined the effect of ginseng on human work capacity and energy by giving ginseng to proof readers and testing their speed and accuracy. Those given ginseng increased the number of letters read by twelve per cent and decreased the mistakes by fifty-one per cent compared with those given a 'mock extract' without ginseng. Another case is reported where young radio operators who had transmitted a radio message were then asked to transmit another long message. Those taking ginseng had a reduction in the mistakes compared with the first trial, despite their tiredness, while those not taking ginseng increased their mistakes.

Reflexes Speed Up
Ginseng stimulates the nervous system itself. Reflexes have been shown to speed up; for example, tests have shown that the eye takes less time to adjust to the dark after taking some. Professor Petkov, of the Institute of Advanced Medical Training in Sofia, has been occupied for the last fifteen years with elaborate experiments to

assess its effects on the nervous system. He finds a typical stimulation of the brain wave patterns (electroéncephelogram) when experimental animals are given ginseng, and has repeatedly observed that the speed of conditioned (learned) reflexes in both animals and human subjects is increased. This implies an increase in efficiency of cerebral activity.

Professor Petkov has also shown the surprising phenomenon that mice which have learned a certain repetitive behaviour pattern and then been allowed to forget it could remember that training after a single low dose of ginseng corresponding to less than 1g for a human. Rats also show an increased mental adaptability, since they can more easily switch from one type of learned response to another when given ginseng. He concludes from these types of experiment that: 'Ginseng stimulates . . . the basic neural processes which constitute the functioning of the cerebral cortex, namely the excitation . . . and inhibition . . . which form the physiological basis of man's mental functioning as a whole.' He continues 'Ginseng, in contrast to other stimulants, causes no disturbance in the equilibrium of the cerebral processes. This explains the absence of any pronounced sense of subjective excitement as is characteristic of all other stimulants . . . and also why this stimulant does not interfere with the normal course of sleep.'

Ginseng as a Sedative

In keeping with its stimulant action on the nervous system, ginseng has been shown to reverse and block the effects of alcohol and sedative drugs such as barbiturates and chlorpromazine. Yet, strangely, it has been demonstrated that there is a sedative component in the root itself. Japanese scientists at the University of Tokyo showed that rats given higher doses of ginseng extract in addition to a sleeping draught slept more and were less restless than with the sleeping draught alone.

How is it possible, one might ask at this point, for a drug to have both a stimulating and a sedative effect? It is indeed possible, and there need be no paradox. It can be shown that ginseng contains a number of components, some of which work in opposite ways. A drug which can have apparently opposite effects is no mystery in traditional medicine. More than that, traditional medicine treasures such drugs, for the value of a single drug which can pick you up if you are tired and sedate you if you are over-excited is obvious. Another feature of the action of ginseng which makes it such a unique medicine is that the more tired you are, the more noticeable will be its effect.

Ginseng Compared with Other Stimulants

As both Professor Petkov and Professor Brekhman have remarked in their reports, there is a world of difference between ginseng and other stimulants such as caffeine or amphetamine.

(a) Ginseng is not an excitant. It does not cause feelings of over-excitation, emotional disturbance or agitation in humans nor, as far as can be judged, in animals.

(b) There is a sedative component in ginseng. Unlike other stimulants, there is no difficulty in sleeping after taking it.

(c) Ginseng acts in a stabilizing fashion. The more tired one is, the more noticeable is its action.
(d) Ginseng causes an increase in health, appetite and mental condition, especially if taken over a period. The other stimulants cause more ill health the longer they are taken.
(e) Ginseng is much safer than other stimulants.
(f) Ginseng may assist in combating stress, while the other stimulants can actually cause stress.

Ginseng and Stress
The body has automatic mechanisms which are called upon if a dangerous or potentially harmful situation arises. Loud noises, threats, wounding, the potential of a wound, fear, anger, emotional tension and so on, all generate the automatic stress response. The response is controlled by hormones. Hormones are chemical substances made in various glands around the body which control and integrate the bodily metabolism and co-ordinate the response of the body to the world outside. They are like nerves, but their message is slower; if nerves are the body's telephone system, then hormones would be the postal service. They govern the stress response, particularly adrenalin, secreted from the adrenal glands. Changes are produced, such as a diversion of blood from the digestive system towards the muscles, muscular tension and heart stimulation.

Many people are under constant stress – for example, today's busy administrators with the telephone ringing, or factory workers who suffer noise and tension on the production line, or people with overwhelming emotional problems. Too much stress is bad for the body. Repeated stimulation of the heart combined with lack of exercise causes cardiovascular problems which are so common in the middle-aged in civilized countries. Digestive troubles and gastric ulcers are also the result of constant outpourings from the adrenal glands. The body becomes tired easily because there is constant arousal and tension in the muscles. The defence mechanism of the body when overworked loses its usefulness and becomes dangerous.

Ginseng has repeatedly been shown to protect the body against stress. Professor Petkov proved that in a group of mice subjected to stress, those taking ginseng showed two basic improvements. Firstly, there was an increase in the weight and function of the adrenal glands, together with less abnormalities of behaviour and distress: the mice were, in fact, more able to 'absorb' stress. One is reminded of the Chinese soldiers who take ginseng with them to the battlefield to help them resist the effects of stress and shock. Secondly, there was an actual *reduction* in the long-term stress response and its corresponding harmful effects. The body had increased its resistance. When ginseng was taken, the animals coped better with actual stress but the body activity settled back to normal more rapidly.

An Adaptogen?
A consideration of the way ginseng can cause resistance to stress leads inevitably to one of the most exciting ideas in pharmacology. Professor Brekhman, and also scientists in South Korea, carried out the following experiments. Mice were given ginseng and subjected to the depressant

action of chloral hydrate, barbiturates and alcohol, and their recovery improved. They were irradiated with X-rays, the most damaging of influences on the body, and their subsequent lifespan was doubled. The mice also showed a greater ability to survive after being given a fiendish collection of poisons and drugs such as potent anti-cancer drugs, after infection with bacteria, and after stress by physical conditions such as heat, cold and change in pressure.

Chemical changes in the body were then measured to see how the mice were coping. The surprising fact is that ginseng had absolutely no effect on these processes in the absence of stress. In other words, it only acted to return the body to normal if it had gone off course. This has led to the exciting concept of using the plant as an 'adaptogen' – a medicine which increased the ability of the body to adapt, and which only works when it is needed. The idea is unique in Western drug research and, apart from ginseng and *Eleutherococcus*, the 'Siberian ginseng', no other drug or medicine is known which has a 'normalizing' effect. To most scientists who have been studying the action of drugs, it would seem hard to believe that such a thing exists. But the evidence is plain for everyone to see and is published in the scientific literature. The Chinese, of course, have recognized this property of ginseng for a long time. They are justified in saying 'I told you so'. A harmless medicine which returns wayward body processes to normal, however mild the effect, may be described as an ideal medicine. The medicine of the past may well turn out to be a medicine of the future.

How can ginseng work as an 'adaptogen'? It is

difficult to know exactly, because it has so many different effects on the body. The secret is likely to be in the way that it acts on the nerves and hormones. The response of the body to the environment is organized by these communication systems. If ginseng improves the efficiency of nerve and hormone messenger systems, then one might expect a greater co-ordination in the defence forces of the body. The body is helped to help itself, whether the problem is abnormally high blood pressure or abnormal tiredness, for example.

There is evidence that ginseng does indeed stimulate several glands to regulate their hormone production, but there is also some evidence against this. One Chinese report states that it acts directly on the adrenal glands to increase the bodily resistance, while a Korean research report states that resistance is improved even when the adrenal glands are removed. We can suggest that some of the actions of ginseng are through hormones, others, as Professor Petkov has shown, are through direct stimulation of the nervous system, and others are by unknown actions directly on the metabolism of body tissues.

What Does Ginseng Contain?
Many of the activities of ginseng have now been positively connected with components called glycosides. Glycosides contain steroids. Many hormones are also steroids. A whole series of glycosides have been isolated by Russian scientists, who called them panaxosides A, B, C and so on. Another series of glycosides, possibly the same ones, has also been isolated by Japanese workers who name them ginsenosides Ra, Rb, Rc.

The difference in the names has, not unexpectedly, led to some confusion for third parties attempting to carry out research into the ginseng components. Besides glycosides the dried ginseng root contains essential oils, fatty acids, ginsenin, phytosterin, mucilaginous resins, enzymes, vitamins, sugars, certain unknown alkaloids, minerals, silicic acid and not more than thirteen per cent moisture.

In this complex mixture of substances one thing stands clear. The glycosides are able to carry out the stimulating and tonic actions of ginseng, and many of its other properties. It is known that different glycosides have slightly different properties. Some are stronger than others when compared in a standard test such as the extra length of time that mice can swim. Professor Shellard at the University of London is occupied in isolating and testing the ginseng glycosides for the purpose of standardizing ginseng preparations. Once a standard is available, it will be possible to tell good ginseng from bad, and additionally to know more accurately the doses being given for different purposes.

There is also evidence that other components of ginseng have alternative activities. Japanese pharmacologists at the University of Tokyo have been able to show that while the water soluble glycosides do indeed have a stimulating effect on the nervous system, alcohol soluble glycosides have an opposite sedative effect and increase the sleeping time of experimental animals.

Other evidence shows that only water soluble glycosides have a stimulatory effect on the metabolism of the body, while only the alcohol soluble steroidal compounds have a sex-hormone type of action. It is clear that there are many components in ginseng which can have different and even contrasting effects. This is a good example of a herb where the whole is greater than its parts.

Ginseng and Disease

A common disability which causes considerable suffering to people, especially those in middle age and above, is cardiovascular disease. It is due to the blockage of blood vessels by fatty deposits and growths and can lead to heart attack when the vessels which are blocked are those supplying blood to the hard-working muscle of the heart itself. When ginseng was given to dogs with artificially induced high blood pressure, the blood pressure was somewhat lowered. Likewise, animals with a sharply reduced blood pressure show, according to Professor Petkov, a small increase. Evidently the adaptogenic action of ginseng includes a moderate stabilizing of the blood pressure.

Cholesterol has been pinpointed as accompanying high blood pressure and blockage of blood vessels. It has been shown that when rabbits are fed on a high cholesterol diet, ginseng included in the diet is able to reduce the level of cholesterol in the body. In clinical trials with elderly patients who had high blood pressure, ginseng was shown to produce a consistent but small reduction in the blood pressure. A German team of doctors reported an average drop of 23 in the blood pressure of patients with a systolic pressure above 140. The Chinese always include ginseng in medicines for those suffering from heart attack or heart disease.

Diabetes is a disturbance of the metabolism of sugar in the liver. Administration of ginseng to animals tends to reduce blood sugar, both in normal animals and those with artificially raised blood sugar. This stabilizing effect is a typical adaptogenic one, since ginseng has also been shown to *raise* blood sugar when it is artificially lowered by insulin injections.

Ginseng has a subtle effect on many different types of metabolism, and research is being carried on at the moment in order to try to understand its action on the chemical processes in the body. Scientists have recently discovered, for example, that it causes a more economical release of body energy and an extra storage of energy-producing compounds in the liver. If animals are forced to take extensive exercise, their supply is not so depleted in the presence of ginseng. The synthesis of proteins in the liver is increased, as is the general rate of 'manufacture' of important body chemicals in the liver cells. It is not certain if these are direct effects of ginseng or the secondary result of the stimulation of the hormone system. Interestingly, ginseng can stimulate the metabolism of body cells even when the cells are isolated and kept in a test tube, so hormones are not always needed for it to work.

Ginseng and Potency
One of the many fabled powers of ginseng is that it increases sexual vitality. Science has something to say about this, namely that ginseng cannot stimulate sexual performance, except in a psychological or suggestive manner. Therefore if it

is believed that it increases sexual prowess, then it probably will, because sexual virility is to some extent a matter of confidence.

Many drugs and medicines have been hopefully called 'aphrodisiacs', but there are in fact very few real aphrodisiacs and it is doubtful if ginseng is one of them. On the other hand, there is scientific evidence that it may have the less notorious but nevertheless important function of helping to restore male potency in some cases of impotence. Many cases of impotence are psychological, but some are due to a decline in the hormones which control the sexual responses. There is clear evidence that ginseng contains compounds with sex hormone activity, and in some experiments it has been shown to reverse harmful effects due to a lack of male sex hormones.

In other experiments the ginseng glycosides were able to encourage the development of the sex organs in young animals. Young mice given ginseng reached puberty faster than untreated mice, and they had prostate glands forty to sixty per cent larger. In fact, the increase in weight of these glands has been suggested by Professor Brekhman as a way of measuring the strength of different ginseng preparations. Dr Karzel of the University of Bonn concludes: 'The occurrence of constituents with sex-hormone-like activity in ginseng preparations thus seems to be proven . . . but questions concerning the ratios between male and female hormones remain to be solved.'

There are clinical reports from Russia of striking improvements when ginseng was given to some patients suffering from sexual impotence. The patients felt more tranquil and active, and showed an improvement in sexual function. Although much more study is needed, we can say that perhaps the Chinese are justified in expecting to be fertile into old age with the help of ginseng.

CHAPTER FIVE

THE ELIXIR?

The Chinese have always been interested in old age. While European alchemists were devoted to the attempt to convert dross into gold, the Chinese alchemists were similarly occupied with finding the elixir of life. The herbal manuals are insistent that ginseng can prolong life, although they recognize that it certainly is not 'The Elixir': 'If even the herb Chu-seng can make one live longer, try putting the Elixir in the mouth' says an alchemical book of A.D. 142.

Of all the people who treasure ginseng in China, it is the old who are most enthusiastic. As we have seen, the common belief is that if taken regularly, it will retard the ageing process, keep crippling diseases such as arthritic and cardiovascular disease at bay, provide energy to old people with flagging vitality, and would even allow men to retain their sexual potency until the very last years of their life. The very best gift that an old man or woman could receive in China would be a good ginseng root.

Much of the lore and ritual concerning the use of ginseng is perpetuated by the elderly. They are the ones who keep ginseng soaking in brandy for years, waiting for the most auspicious occasion to consume it; who respect ginseng for its supposed radiation and keep it in lead-lined boxes; who will spend their life's savings on select roots. Mao Tse-Tung and Chou en-Lai are both known to take ginseng regularly. Father Jartoux was also in complete agreement with the Chinese belief that ginseng was able to prolong life and wrote enthusiastically about it.

The Ageing Process

Can ginseng really help a man to resist the effects of ageing? This is really two questions. Is such a thing as a 'Fountain of Youth' possible? If so, would ginseng qualify as one? In order to answer these questions we have to know something more about the ageing process.

Ageing is inevitable. Despite the biblical statement that Methusaleh and others lived many hundreds of years, it is accepted that the potential lifespan is strictly limited to about 100 years. Well before this time the body begins to run down. The correct working of the organs, the cells, the bodily metabolism slowly deteriorates. Scientists have recently demonstrated that the very information which controls the construction and smooth running of the body wears itself out, just like the message on a tape will become obscured after many re-runs through a tape recorder. This is the *process* of ageing, but there is an important difference between the process of ageing and the *effect* of ageing.

As ageing continues, the body becomes more and more vulnerable to disease and damage. Old people are increasingly likely to catch infections, for example, or they tend to have slower reactions and are therefore more likely to be involved in a road accident.

Resisting the Effects of Ageing

The *process* of ageing cannot be altered or manipulated by any external agent. Scientists admit that a real elixir of life is not foreseeable. Immortality is a myth and it will remain so. This is not so gloomy as it sounds, because the *effects* of ageing can be mollified. The motto of the American Gerontological Society is 'To Add Life to Years not Years to Life'.

Supposing it were possible to so increase the resistance of the body that despite ageing continuing at its own pace, no premature illnesses were suffered by the old person. In that case the person would reach his potential lifespan. He would be healthy and active right until the day he died. He would just 'die of old age' when his body could not function any more. Country people in some Shangri-La areas of the world – secluded valleys in the mountains of South Russia, Hunza in Pakistan, Villacamba in Ecuador – have a large number of very old people who are healthy and are reaching their maximum potential lifespan. It may be 100 years or just over.

In general, any treatment that improves the health and fitness of the body can be expected to assist in resisting the effects of ageing, despite the ageing process itself continuing at the same rate. Yoga and exercise can both have an effect on the lifespan in this way. Alternatively, cigarette smoking can shorten the lifespan by making the body more vulnerable to cancer and bronchial infections.

Every culture has traditional remedies and treatments which are purported to lead to a healthy long life. In the West a proliferation of possible substances has been in the news, such as Vitamin C, Vitamin E, unsaturated oils in food, procaine, anti-oxidants (similar to food preservatives!) and synthetic hormones. In addition, comfrey root, liquorice, garlic and vegetarian food are traditional suggestions.

In India there is a special section of traditional medicine, called *Rasaaynen*, which is devoted to resisting the effects of ageing. This treatment is of great antiquity and complexity. It involves an elaborate series of herbs which are to be taken over a long period while the subject is living inside a specially built room or cell, the precise measurements of which are laid down. Some noted Indian politicians, such as Jawaharlal Nehru, are known to have undergone this process.

The Chinese, of course, have a rich source of different herbal medicines which are useful in combating ageing symptoms, but none of the same repute as ginseng. One Peking professor, reported the *New York Times* in 1933, lived for 256 years. He attributed his purported longevity to a tea that he brewed daily. The tea contained ginseng and '*Fo ti teng*', which is *Hydrocotyle asiatica*, a common creeping plant.

In the early 'twenties, Claude Bernard, a distinguished scientist, introduced a fashion for eating the gonads of monkeys as a way of prolonging life. Scientists at that time believed that ageing was due to the failure of the hormones of the body and that taking hormones in the form of monkey glands could slow down the process.

A rather less crude development of hormone therapy arrived with the availability of synthetic hormones such as testosterone. Testosterone is still taken nowadays, although only in special cases of premature impotence or decline in vitality. It has certain harmful side effects with prolonged use.

In theory, hormone therapy could slow down some of the effects of ageing, because the efficiency of the internal hormones does indeed decline with age. Taking hormones will compensate but only for a limited period.

Ginseng and Ageing

The Chinese find European involvement with monkey glands amusing. Why, they ask, does one need to eat monkey glands when a natural plant exists which is much more effective, longer lasting and safer? The intriguing fact is that ginseng also seems to act very much like a hormone, but in addition stimulates the body to produce its own hormones. This may be one way in which it could moderate the effects of ageing.

We have also seen how a decline in resistance is a key manifestation of ageing. Ginseng is almost the only known substance which can increase bodily resistance. One of the major effects of ageing, especially in the developed countries, is a degeneration of the blood system causing strokes, heart attacks, etc. We know that ginseng helps to treat cardiovascular diseases and diabetes. Another common complaint of the elderly is tiredness, and we have demonstrated that ginseng is a safe and effective long term stimulant. All these factors would suggest that ginseng is ideal for treatment of the symptoms of ageing.

There is unfortunately very little scientific evidence on this aspect of ginseng. It would be difficult to demonstrate an effect on the lifespan of humans, because it would take so long that the scientists themselves would be old at the end of the experiment.

Animals can be used, however; the lifespan of a mouse is two years. Observations on the effect of ginseng on the lifespan of mice are being carried out at this moment in the University of London. The treated mice appeared more active and energetic, but it will take another year to know if their lifespan is affected.

It is also possible to carry out experiments on human cells isolated from the body. Ginseng has been shown by the author and other scientists to stimulate the growth of such cells, and to delay the death and disintegration of the cells under inhospitable conditions. Such experiments are just the beginning.

Tests Just Beginning

Trials of ginseng with old people in hospitals and old-age homes are also just getting off the ground. They have already given encouraging results. In one case, sixty-six patients in the age range thirty to sixty were given ginseng and vitamins. Improvements were noticed in most of the patients who suffered from cardiovascular diseases, depression and reduced vitality. There were also psychological benefits. Many of the patients revealed an awakening of interest in life. The psychological aspects are also the most marked feature of another recent clinical trial. Two German doctors gave ginseng to ninety-five patients in old-age homes. Besides improvements in blood pressure, memory, neurological function and bodily function, fifty-eight of the patients showed 'an enhancement of mood so marked as to be almost euphoric, and in almost all cases it was maintained for a period of months'. The doctors then continue: 'It goes without saying that tiredness or exhaustion was one of our patients main symptoms ... 83% showed clear improvements in both these syndromes, which can be considered an excellent result.'

It may be true to say that ginseng is ideal for old people. It is my belief that the Chinese have introduced to the world the only drug or medicine which has ever been shown to have medicinal powers which specifically fit the conditions of the elderly. Others who have researched into ginseng also hold this view. Professor Brekhman has been claiming for many years that ginseng would be of great interest to gerontologists (those studying ageing). One international company has been marketing a geriatric preparation for some time which is widely available in Europe. Its main constituent is ginseng.

Not an Elixir

A note of caution is necessary. It can be dangerous to raise false hopes. We have shown that ginseng cannot be regarded as an elixir. It can only palliate the effects of ageing. Even this it does in a mild and gentle manner, building up over a long period. Like many other herbs, it works gradually and the effects are not violent and dramatic. Moreover, it cannot be expected to cure the degenerative diseases of old age. It is likely to produce a mild improvement, but its main function would be to help the body resist developing these conditions in the first place. For this purpose it must be taken continuously and regularly. It is well known that people vary considerably in their response to drugs and herbs and the effects of ginseng may or may not be immediately noticeable depending on other factors such as diet, the quality of the root and so on.

There are other ways in which old people could maximize the chances of attaining a healthy old age, which are probably in the long run more effective than any tonics, including ginseng. Diet should be moderate, with plenty of roughage, fresh fruit and vegetables or grains, avoiding fatty and rich foods, sugar and starch. Exercise should be regular and sufficiently vigorous, and should be maintained throughout life because it is difficult and even dangerous to begin vigorous exercise in advanced age. Stress-free living, a sanguine and calm existence, is essential to health. This includes an intelligent avoidance of harmful environmental influences.

CHAPTER SIX

HOW TO TAKE GINSENG

Both the claims made for ginseng by the Chinese and the experiments of modern science can be used for a practical purpose: to inform those who are interested in taking ginseng how to take it. The following are the uses for which ginseng can be recommended.

(a) *Stimulant*. Ginseng has been shown to be a safe, effective and natural stimulant with many advantages over other stimulants such as caffeine or amphetamines. It can be taken for tiredness and exhaustion, or when going through a heavily taxing task, such as examinations, long-distance driving, stage performances, unusually strenuous physical work and so on. It is ideally suited for those occasions when one is exhausted from overwork, insomnia or over-indulgence, and may be a very effective way of coping with a hangover. In these cases it should be taken at the time when it is needed. The doses are given on page 55.

(b) *Tonic*. The Chinese tend to pay more attention to ginseng as a long-term restorative, because it is believed that benefits to health only accrue from the gradual and continuous use of natural medicines. It is recommended in convalescence from disease, in coping with long-term tiredness, in removing the feeling of being below par ('one degree under'). Taking ginseng at these times may not only remove the feeling of being off colour and tired, but also decrease the likelihood of incurring a disease due to lowered bodily resistance. It may also be taken for diseases such as anaemia and dysentery, where tiredness is a side effect.

(c) *Mental benefits*. Judging from the Russian experience with ginseng for improving the mental state of the elderly, there are also psychological benefits to be obtained from its long-term use. It can be recommended for depression and insomnia, as it has been documented repeatedly that it is able to raise spirits and improve outlook on life, especially among the elderly. Its general tonic effects may also assist memory and concentration.

(d) *Anti-stress*. Ginseng taken regularly may assist in coping with the stresses and strains of life. It may also help the body resist the harmful long-term effect of stress which, as we have seen, can produce damaging changes to the blood system and the digestion.

(e) *Regulating blood pressure*. Although it has been demonstrated to have a mild stabilizing effect on blood pressure, whether low or high, the causes of irregular blood pressure are often inherent changes in the cardiovascular system, and they cannot actually be reversed or cured by ginseng. It can safely be taken as a regular course by those with disorders of the cardiovascular system, but it should be on a trial and error basis, and with the full knowledge and consent of the individual's doctor. Ginseng can be taken in addition to any other drugs which may have been prescribed, without risk of incompatibility.

(f) *Anti-diabetic*. As there is some evidence that ginseng can adjust the blood sugar level in cases of diabetes, it may be taken by diabetics, and if there is a noticeable improvement this can be taken into account in the long-term management of the disease. Again, there will be no problems of incompatibility with other treatments as the herb is mild and extremely safe. It is better to be dependent on ginseng to assist in the management of a particular disease – if it helps – than to be dependent on stronger allopathic medicines.

(g) *Against impotence.* This is an area of treatment full of 'quackery' and old wives' tales. As we have seen, impotence may be psychological rather more often than physical, and ginseng may help certain cases of physical impotence, particularly where it is the result of a general lack of vitality. Chinese doctors have placed great faith in long-term courses of ginseng for the treatment of physical impotence, and especially the decline in potency which accompanies ageing. Incidentally, the Chinese say that when it is used for the treatment of flagging vitality (both sexual and otherwise), it should be accompanied by a period of continence. They believe that continence will cause secretions which arise through the use of ginseng to become reabsorbed into the blood stream and thus revitalize the brain and the body. The herb is not an aphrodisiac, i.e. a substance to be taken at the time of sexual activity to increase virility.

(g) *Health in old age.* This has been dealt with fully in Chapter Five. Suffice it to say here that for this purpose ginseng must be taken regularly – at least one course a year. The frequency of consumption should increase with age, so that after middle age some is taken every day.

The Way to Take Ginseng

The rituals in China concerned with the consumption of ginseng are as great as those of gathering or cultivation, but almost any convenient way of ingesting it would be medically acceptable. Much of the ginseng in China is boiled and extracted for long periods with water, or water and alcohol, to give a dark extract which is sold commercially in a number of closely related forms. Drops of extract are then taken neat or dripped into tea. Ginseng can also be chewed: a nugget of the required size is cut from the root, or a ready prepared ball of ginseng coated in wax is purchased and the piece chewed thoroughly until it is completely soft. Another popular method is to boil the root to make a tea. Special silver kettles are used for this purpose, because it is a hard and fast rule that no other metal apart from silver can come into contact with the root. The general tradition is to boil it for between six and ten hours, starting in the evening, then get up at dawn, drink the preparation and go back to sleep. It is also common, especially among old people, to take a whole root, together with some leaves if possible, and put it in a bottle of brandy. This is then stored for a long time, after which glasses are taken regularly with the greatest relish!

Any of these methods of consumption would be suitable for those in the West, depending on the types of root available. Root pieces and whole roots are sometimes available in health food shops, and Chinese stores will certainly stock them. The more expensive red roots are mostly only available in Chinese shops, since the ginseng exported to European pharmaceutical and health goods distribution companies is all white ginseng, mostly from Korea and occasionally China. Root pieces and whole roots can be chewed thoroughly or boiled. Powdered root makes a palatable tea. Extract is also widely available in Europe. Some companies make it in Europe from imported roots, and sell it with or without the addition of vitamins. Korean suppliers also export ready prepared packets of 'instant ginseng tea' made from the root, and sometimes from the leaf or the flower of the plant. These drinks are tasty but of reduced medicinal potency compared with the root or extract. The enterprise of the Korean manufacturers is hard to believe. In Korean supermarkets today one can buy ginseng candies, ginseng chewing gum, ginseng hair lotion, ginseng creams and cosmetics, and even ginseng soup flavourings!

How Safe is Ginseng?

It has already been mentioned that ginseng is remarkably safe, even in large doses, or when taken over a long period, and modern research has confirmed this. Professor Brekhman writes that a harmful dose for animals has been shown to be at least 1000 times the effective dose – equivalent to a man eating three to four pounds of pure ginseng at one sitting. More recently, Professor Savel of the Pharmaceutical faculty of Paris University has tried to give sufficient ginseng to mice to cause side effects. He failed: the mice suffered from enlarged stomachs due to overeating but were otherwise well.

Italian scientists gave large doses of ginseng to mice continuously for six months without any noticeable ill effects, and clinical trials with patients have never shown any harmful side effects. In the Kaschenko hospital in Russia, patients were undergoing ginseng treatment for depression and other psychiatric disturbances. The doctors noticed a general improvement, but with six patients 'sexual excitement was found to have been produced as a side effect'. A decision on whether this is a harmful or beneficial side effect will have to be left to the reader.

Dosage

The label on a packet of ginseng may describe a recommended dose. How reliable are these instructions? How much of the root should one take? Are there any differences in the doses for different purposes? We can be guided in these questions by a synthesis of the Chinese traditional usage with its thousands of years of experience and the careful analysis of modern science.

The Chinese chew pieces of ginseng varying in size from a pea to a walnut, and they would take more than one such piece a day. This would correspond to between two and six grams of root a day, and is also the recommended dose in the *Pharmacopoeia Japonica*, but is about twice as much as is usually recommended in European preparations. This may be because the Chinese are more confident about ginseng than the Europeans. Indeed, the amounts taken by the Chinese sometimes seem to be dictated by how much they can afford rather than any other considerations. Moreover, the quality of the Chinese root is probably somewhat better than the root commonly available in the West, which would make the actual difference in dosage even greater. The herbal books and sources generally prescribe a dosage of approximately two grams of root a day to be taken every day for a considerable period.

Scientific experiments have shown that mice are noticeably stimulated by a dose of ginseng which would be equivalent to five grams for an adult human. On the other hand, mice are not so sensitive to drugs as humans, and in human trials as little as one-fifth of a gram has been shown to have a noticeably arousing effect. The dosages used in experiments vary. The equivalent of three grams in extract form was given to the radio operators in the experiment by Professor Brekhman described in Chapter Four.

In conclusion, we can recommend that to build up vitality and for all long-term uses, between half and one gram should be taken twice a day. The course should last for at least a month and preferably two months. Older people can take ginseng continuously at a total dose of one or two grams a day. For a short-term effect, i.e. as a stimulant, to combat fatigue and exhaustion, and in cases of weakness during convalescence, the dose may be increased somewhat. Two or three grams a day will be sufficient, again divided into a dose in the morning and in the evening.

Varying Effects

It is a common experience that some people notice the effects of ginseng and others do not. In general, most people notice a stimulation with higher doses, but this depends on whether they are exhausted or not. The more exhausted they are, the more they will notice a return to normality. During the long-term use of ginseng in lower doses, people may or may not be conscious of any change. This is because there are enormous constitutional differences in the way people respond to drugs. Thinner people, for example, tend to be more sensitive to drugs, as do those used to a simple diet. Someone on a frugal diet may notice the effects of ginseng more than someone who eats meat and rich foods.

There are also psychological factors at work. Some people believe that ginseng has such a strong effect that taking a reasonable dose makes them 'high'. It has become fashionable among the young people on the west coast of America to consume quantities of the root throughout the day for this purpose. A German newspaper reported in September 1974 that a young man walked into a Berlin pharmacy brandishing a gun and demanded two packets of ginseng. He must have wanted it badly!

Ginseng is no more 'an alternative to pot and alcohol', as one sensation-seeking news article claims, than is garlic. On the other hand, it can undoubtedly generate a feeling of health and vitality and therefore a sense of well-being. Some people get the same feeling from a sauna bath, but it would be an exaggeration to say that a sauna bath makes people high. It can be stated categorically that there are no grounds for suggesting that ginseng has any intoxicating effect. On the contrary, it has been shown to protect the body from intoxication by alcohol and other drugs. It would thus be more accurate to say that ginseng 'helps you recover from pot and alcohol'.

CHAPTER SEVEN

GINSENG AND TRADITIONAL MEDICINE TODAY

It has taken literally thousands of years for ginseng to appear in shops in the West. Doctors are not generally familiar with it, and those who are often regard it as 'yet another useless fad'. The climate of medical opinion has hardly changed from that put forward in the Smithsonian Institute report at the beginning of the century: 'Ginseng has no value as far as Western medicine can judge ... its effects being purely psychological ... but we have only scratched the surface of Chinese medical knowledge.'

Only a few years ago top medical experts of the West were saying exactly the same thing about acupuncture: that it had no real value, that it was mere trickery or hypnotism. They were often so scathing in their condemnation that practitioners were hardly differentiated from witches. Now the same experts have completely reversed their opinion and recognize it as a technique that has great potential usefulness. It must be said that no one in the West has yet published any report which really understands acupuncture. One might suggest that, like the apparently paradoxical aspects of ginseng, it will be hard to understand if one tries to approach it from a conventional point of view. It needs to be seen from the viewpoint of traditional medicine and the Chinese view of the body and its ailments.

Why Has Ginseng Been Ignored?

It is quite possible that ginseng will follow the same road as acupuncture. It may one day be recognized as an important new aid to health and become widely used in the West. Then the question might be raised: why is it that such an obviously beneficial substance has been ignored for so long? Several reasons can be suggested:

1. The experience of the first people to study ginseng 'has not been based on the true plant which is difficult to get and costly' wrote C. F. Leyel, F.R.S. This resulted in a self-perpetuating myth that the herb was useless, which was passed from one expert to the next and recorded in reports and such books as *Encyclopaedia Britannica*.

2. Large numbers of reports have been published on ginseng in the scientific journals of China, Russia, Japan and Korea. There may be as many as 500. Yet most of these are without translation, and very few have been read by Western scientists. This is partly because of the difficulty of getting hold of the reports, but mostly because there has been very little interest among experts for such information from the East. The flow of information on medicine and science has been mostly in one direction – from West to East. Apart from an 'information gap', there is also a 'credibility gap', so that even when some information does arrive in the West, it is often ignored or treated with suspicion, for the experts involved trust neither the authors whom they do not know, nor the journal which they do not respect.

3. Western medicines are mostly synthetic and are strictly standardized, manufactured, packaged

and distributed by a large pharmaceutical industry with a powerful voice in medicine. Doctors feel that unless a medicine is of this category it should not be used. Their attitude has probably been formed by their training in medical schools, and by the advertisements of the pharmaceutical industry. The pharmaceutical industry is strongly opposed to natural medicines, because it could not support itself on the distribution of herbs and roots.

4. Ginseng, like many other herbs, has a subtle and mild effect, which is most beneficial when the root is taken regularly for a period. There is also no specific disease that can be said to be *cured* by ginseng. All the effects that have been discussed in the preceding pages are so different from conventional medicines that if comparisons are made with powerful synthetic drugs ginseng may be regarded as inconsequential. There are also some features, such as its 'adaptogenic' power, which are puzzling if regarded from a conventional point of view. Ginseng has been thought about in the past in a way calculated to miss its most advantageous features.

Synthetic Drugs versus Plant Drugs

The strange fact is that although many doctors regard herbalists and naturopaths as not far from quacks, large numbers of synthetic medicines used by doctors are originally derived from plants. The medicines may have been extracted, altered and resynthesized for the purpose of standardization and so on, but often the original discovery and isolation of the drug was made through traditional herbs: digitalis, the important heart-stabilizing glycoside from the foxglove; morphine from the poppy; quinine, once vital in the treatment of malaria, from the bark of a tree; reserpine, used in the treatment of mental disease, from raowolfia; the list is endless.

Perhaps it is not so widely known that much research is still going on to find newer and newer medicines from traditional plant remedies. Very recently, the powerful plant anti-cancer alkaloids vinblastine and vincristine were found in the plant *Vinca rosea*, which has been used since ancient times in Indian medicine. The United States' multi-million dollar drive against cancer includes a new and massive survey of medicinal plants used in traditional medicine for their possible anti-cancer properties. No one would argue that the pharmaceutical industry was founded on plants.

It would therefore be more accurate to say that the medical world is opposed to plants which have not yielded chemically defined and standardized chemicals, rather than against plants as such. As one eminent British scientist said about ginseng: 'It is no use doing any research on it until we know what it contains.' This attitude is precisely that which prevents Western medical experts from understanding and utilizing the wealth of traditional medicines. Who cares what chemicals are inside the plant, as long as it works safely? There is no point in forgetting the aims of medicine in favour of extracting and synthesizing drugs.

Besides ignoring some important medicines which happen to be too complicated to yield known active ingredients, there is a more serious danger. The process of extracting and defining the active principle may leave out other constituents which are present in the plant and are important for a balanced treatment.

The herbalist understands that medicines must be as subtly balanced as music. Extraction of only one component is like throwing out all the instruments in an orchestra except the loudest. Not only is this unnecessary, it may actually be harmful. For example, aspirin was extracted from willow in the seventeenth century. It was probably the first medicine to be purified and synthesized. After 300 years of constant use, it has now been shown to cause side effects such as stomach bleeding. It would have been better not to use it in such a concentrated and purified form.

Ginseng is one of the few herbs for which there is clear scientific evidence that there are more medicinal powers in the entire plant than in any of the chemicals so far isolated from it.

Multiple and Paradoxical Uses

Conventional scientific research, in attempting to extract a single chemical, also looks for a single defined action of a drug. For example, tests will be carried out to see if a drug can raise the blood pressure, or lower the blood pressure. Ginseng is unique because it seems to be one of the first herbs for which there is scientific evidence that the whole root can have multiple and apparently paradoxical effects. It can both raise and lower the blood pressure, or act as a stimulant and a sedative. Allopathic medicine would prefer one defined drug to raise the blood pressure and another drug to lower it, neither of which drugs could adjust to the body's requirements as ginseng does. This shows that the very philosophy behind conventional medicine needs to be brought up to date.

It would be foolish to go to the opposite extreme and become prejudiced against conventional medicine. There are, of course, a multitude of things that the more powerful synthetic medicines can do that herbs cannot. One need only think of the new drugs available which can now eliminate tuberculosis, leprosy and malaria, or the vaccines which can completely protect a person from catching smallpox or cholera, or the injections which can keep a diabetic in relatively perfect health. My purpose is to point out that there are gaps in conventional medicine which can be very successfully filled by 'natural medicine'. Herbal medicines should be used alongside conventional medicine as in China. The herbs should be used to maintain health, as restoratives and tonics, while the stronger medicines should be used, as mentioned in the Emperor Shen Nung's *Pharmacopoeia of the Heavenly Husbandman*, when a serious illness occurs despite all the other efforts. This would be 'the best of the old and the new'.

Ginseng is being used a little more widely every day. It is already sold in the health food shops in many European countries, and is the main constituent in the only widely available geriatric preparation on sale in Europe. We can expect that as it gets more widely known, serious research might begin in the West on its properties. Doctors might know more about it and prescribe courses of it to increase the health of their patients, as they do in Russia and China.

In the United Kingdom, ginseng is not readily accepted by the medical profession. This is illustrated by a recent recommendation that no advertisements should be allowed to make any claim whatsoever for it. On the other hand, there are many enthusiasts who take ginseng, including some doctors and psychiatrists. It is often in the news. Henry Kissinger, who skipped around the world with such energy, was in the news because of his possession of ginseng; so were the North Vietnamese. In fact, during the long hours of the Paris peace conference on Vietnam, the North Vietnamese delegation were never apparently tired or exhausted. When questioned about this by the other diplomats, they produced some ginseng with a flourish.

The last word should come from Sir Edwin Arnold, the famous translator, traveller and author, who eloquently sums up the case for ginseng as a result of his experience in China:

> According to the Chinese, Asiatic ginseng is the best and most potent of all cordials, stimulants, tonics, stomachics, cardiacs, febrifuges, and above all, will best renovate and invigorate failing forces. It fills the heart with hilarity, while its occasional use will, it is said, add a decade to human life. Can all these generations of Orientals who have praised heaven for ginseng's many benefits have been totally deceived? Was humanity ever quite mistaken when half of it believed in something never puffed and never advertised?